T0054249

The Joy Of
BOOBIES

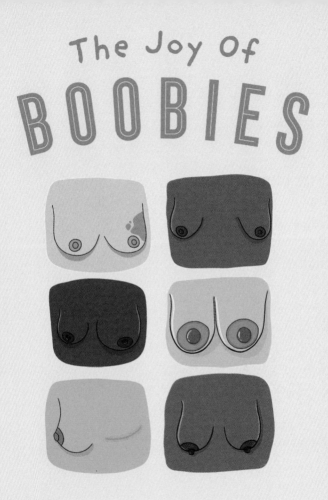

HarperCollins*Publishers*

Introduction

All boobs were created equal. Whether you have little boobs (and don't even need to wear a bra), or boobs so large that you need some serious upholstery to keep them off your belly, each and every type of breast should be celebrated.

The true beauty of breasts is that they are yours to do with as you choose. You can embellish the girls with piercings, tattoos or tassels, or let them be to find their own path. You might show them off to all and sundry or keep them private. Perhaps you have said goodbye to yours or maybe you have created some that you weren't gifted at birth. However your journey has led you to where you are now, or whatever journey of self-love you are still on, it's important to remember that each breast is unique and special, and tells a story.

Sadly, not all of us are perfectly happy with what's on our chest, either because our breasts are no longer what they once were, or they're not what society has conditioned us to think are the ideal shape. But this 'ideal' is so rare it's almost a myth, sported by pretty much only models and anyone else confident enough to flash their knockers on a regular basis. Visibility is everything, so the aim of this book is to demonstrate — in full colour — the large variety of breasts that exist out there, all equally valid and significant. All hail the all-powerful tits!

You will hopefully find yourself reflected here, at least in part. The aim is to be as inclusive as possible and any oversight is unintentional. Gender non-binary and trans* people (the asterisk used to reflect the broad community of individuals) may use different words to describe what's on their chests, so if you're in an intimate relationship with someone who identifies this way and it feels appropriate, you should ask them what term they prefer to use.

Little boobs

With these cute li'l breasts you know the true joys in life — going braless, sleeping on your front, going for a run without needing military-grade support or buying bras with the sole aim of looking nice. You lucky thing!

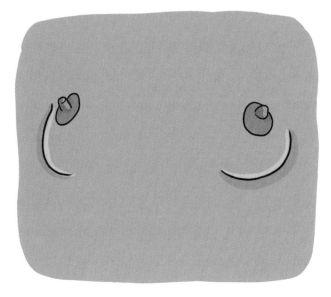

Medium-sized boobs

Just because your boobs lie somewhere in the middle, don't let anyone tell you they're only 'average'. The perfect handful, these breasts are perfectly peachy, clothes hang nicely off them and you're always going to find the bra you want in your size.

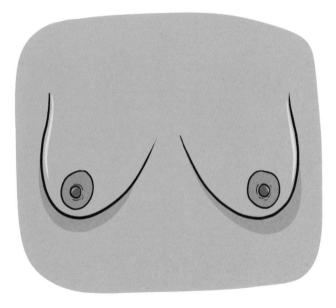

Big boobs

Wear these beauties proud!
Large, round and bouncy,
you make an impact when
you enter a room — but just
remember, they're merely
your warm-up act, so don't let
them define you, or alter your
behaviour because of them.
You are always going to be
the main event.

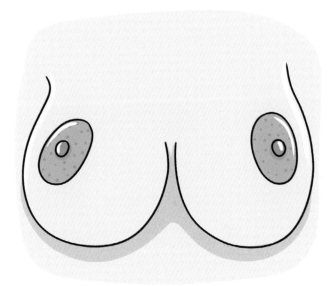

ENORMOUS
boobs

Also known as 'melons' or
'Pamelas' (after the Baywatch
bombshell), these babies may
cause you backache if you don't
invest in a decent bra. You may
also get a little tired of hearing
never-ending compliments on
them (particularly when they're
most certainly not invited), but
your mammoth melons do make a
handy shelf for a cup of tea.

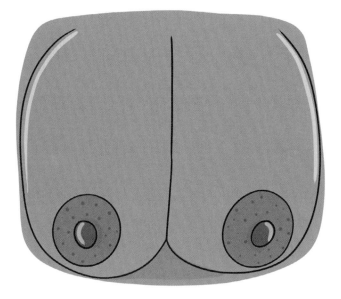

Uneven boobs

Some women feel a little embarrassed by having different-sized breasts, but we should all take comfort in the fact that we form a pretty large club. More than half of us have some variation in the size of our knockers (with the left usually the bigger party, in an unexplained quirk of nature). A bra padded on one side disguises this in the wild, but there's no shame in some irregularity!

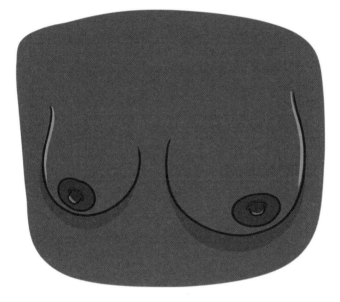

Asymmetrical boobs

These are breasts that are different shapes (rather than necessarily different sizes), but we feel the old adage for eyebrows also works here: 'They should be sisters, not twins.' Whoever wanted boobs that are exactly identical anyway? Variety is the spice of life.

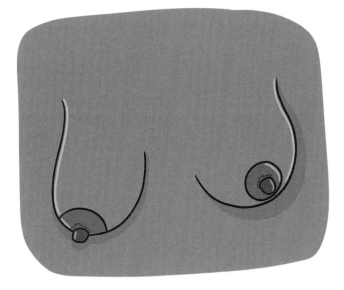

Enhanced boobs

Some women are naturally
blessed with boobs they're
happy with, while others pay
to get them looking the way they
want. Enhanced boobs may look
and feel different, but with a
good surgeon you may find no
one would ever guess. There is
no wrong path to self-love and
however we reach it, let's just all
be pleased if we can get there.

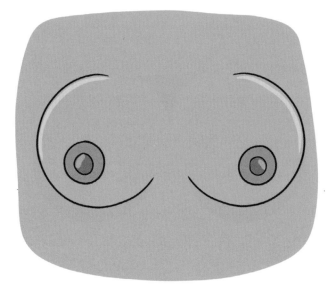

Reduced boobs

To anyone without extremely large breasts, surgery to decrease their size might seem hard to understand — and you may be met with many opinions on the subject. But for many this option is incredibly liberating, both physically and mentally, and the new, smaller breasts can completely change your life.

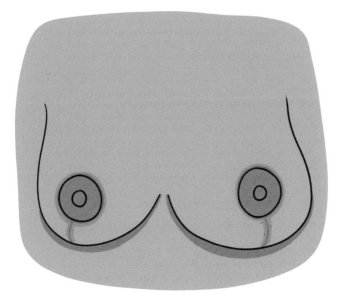

Wide boobs

Also called 'canoes', these girls
are wider horizontally than they
are tall and they stretch across
your chest to create a little
ledge. If you're so inclined to
offer them in this way, they
make the perfect pillow for
someone seeking a comforting
place to rest their head.

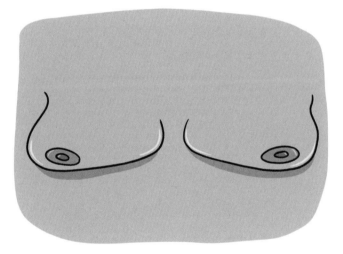

Long boobs

Typically longer and narrower
than other boobs, these tits
do a great pendulum swing and
look great in a plunge bra.

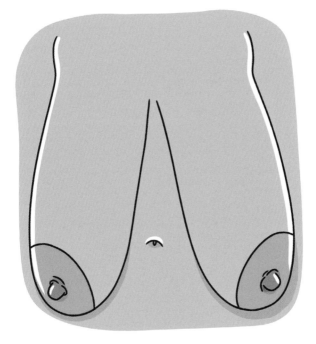

Peachy boobs

Most common in younger women, these pert, gravity-defying puppies are the kind a lot of women dream of. Sadly, they are nowhere near as common as everyone might think and are unlikely to last for ever. If you are blessed with them, enjoy them, but don't be too dismayed if after a few years they start to take the almost-inevitable journey south for the winter.

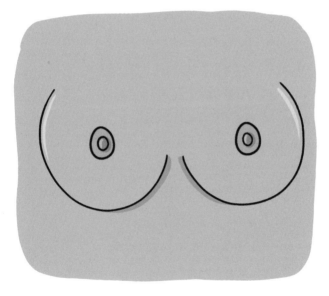

Athletic boobs

You don't have to be an athlete to have this boob-type, but they are most common in those who work out. Wider, with more muscle and less breast tissue than other breast types, they're perfectly adapted to someone who wants to run the hurdles without being knocked out by a rogue mammary on the way. (But whatever your breast type, do get yourself a good sports bra for when you're getting active.)

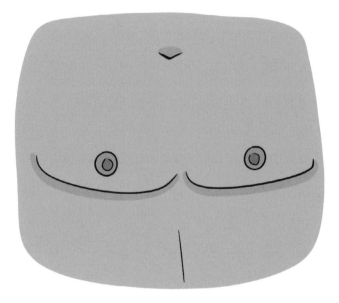

Relaxed boobs

These elongated boobs typically have looser breast tissue. They can occur at any age but most likely later in life, for those who don't wear bras or after weight loss or breastfeeding. In the latter case, many women describe them as being like deflated balloons once the milk has gone — but whatever they look like, they are truly remarkable and should be celebrated for the tireless service they have performed.

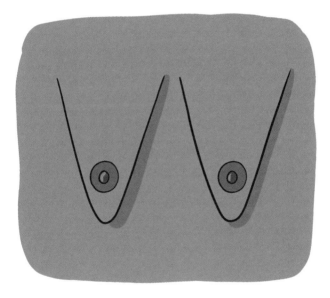

Round boobs

Just as full on top as they are
underneath, these breasts are
unlikely to change shape when
you're doing a handstand.

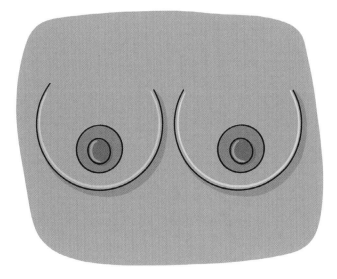

Bell-shaped
boobs

As the name suggests, these
breasts resemble a bell with
a narrow top and a rounder
bottom. Typically occurring in
women with larger breasts,
they may receive the odd 'ding-
dong!' from admirers.

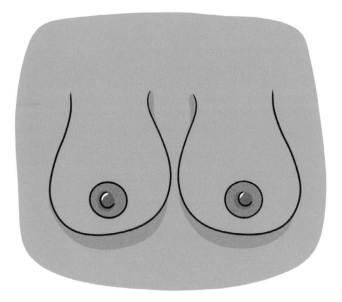

Tear-drop boobs

Sometimes confused with the bell shape, the main difference is that the tear drop is rounder and slightly fuller on the bottom than the top. The name, it should be noted, is entirely reflective of the shape of the breast and no indication that having them would be likely to cause weeping — they are lovely breasts to have.

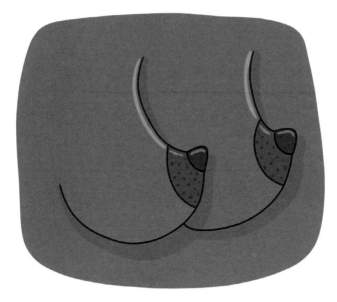

Conical boobs

Also known as 'the Marilyn's'
or simply 'pointy', conical
boobs were extremely en vogue
in the forties and fifties,
accentuated by the 'bullet bra'.
This shape is more commonly
found on smaller boobs.

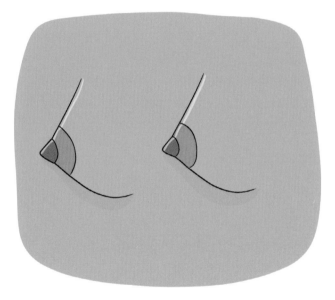

Close-set boobs

Whether you have a small or large bust, these boobs are characterised by how close together they sit on your chest. Great for party tricks (demonstrating all the objects you can hold up with the strength of your breasts), you also have some pretty impressive permanent cleavage (just beware of long necklaces, which will likely get lost).

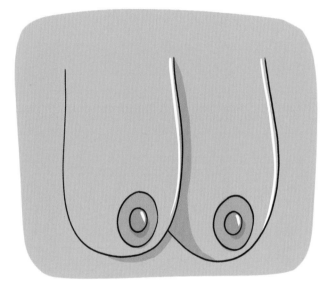

Far-apart boobs

These boobs sit further apart from one another, making cleavage more tricky, but they do give a great side boob aspect. They also make it much more comfortable for you to sleep on your front — win-win!

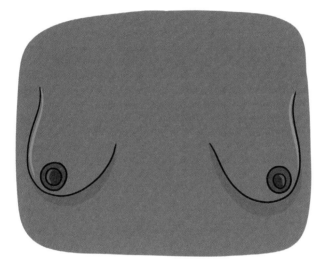

East-West boobs

Whether close together or far apart, this boob type is characterised by the direction your nipples point — away from one another. Also known as 'the divorce' or the 'snobs', we like to think they're not so much estranged from one another as simply pursuing their own interests.

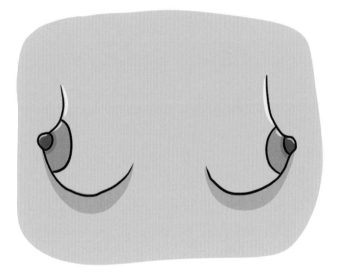

Watch-where-you're-going boobs

These nips are always straining to see what's going on around your feet, drawn down to point southwards. Sadly, there's no evidence yet to suggest this helps prevent you from tripping over things or falling flat on your face.

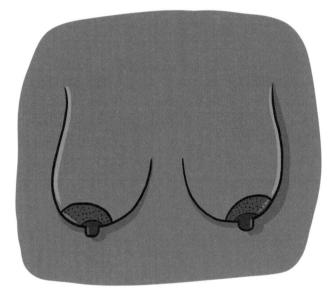

Tiny-nipple boobs

Very neat and proper, this boob type has itsy-bitsy nipples balanced politely atop your breasts. They make wearing skimpy bikinis much easier, but don't worry — it won't take prospective lovers much longer to locate them than more average-sized nips.

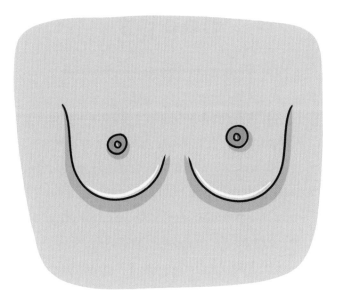

Large-nipple boobs

Nipples and areolas come in all shapes and sizes, and yours are just bigger than most. Sexy as anything, these large nips can be like bullseyes to potential partners, and hopefully you can appreciate your immense mammillas for the works of art that they truly are.

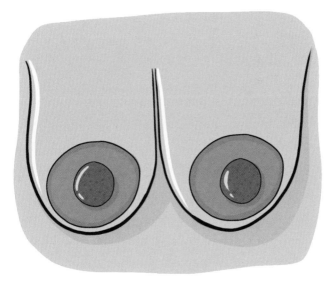

Introverted boobs

If you have inverted nipples, it means the nipple is pulled inward into the breast, remaining flat or concave and refusing to become erect on its own. Some people are born with them, while others develop them later in life. They are certainly no cause for concern and although some women worry about breastfeeding, there is usually no issue.

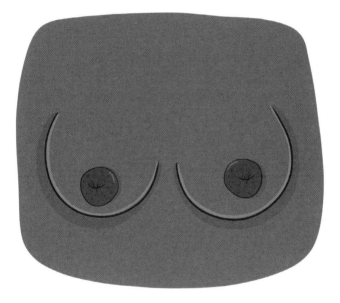

Bound chest

Breasts aren't for everyone and chest-binding is common among anyone who doesn't want their chest to look feminine or is waiting for surgery to remove them. As long as it's done safely, it is a wonderfully liberating practice for trans men, gender non-binary and genderfluid people. There is also a long history of chest-binding in other cultures (such as in Japan) as well as among drag-king performers. It was also used by 1920s' flapper girls hoping to achieve a less traditional look.

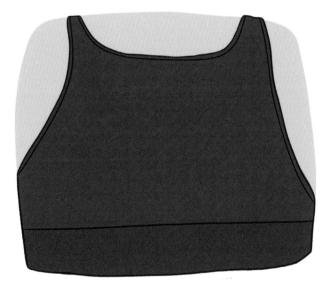

Breast-form boobs

For trans women wanting to dial up the femininity in their day-to-day lives, synthetic breasts can be the perfect way to customise what's on your chest. With so many options out there, including many of the shapes in this book, it's time to herald that dream silhouette.

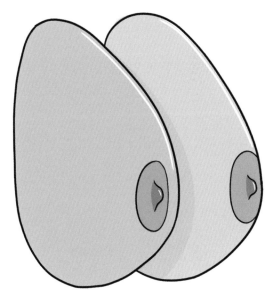

New boobs

Welcome to the boob club!
We hope you love your new
boobs because they look fab.
(Although, of course, with
or without the surgery, we
recognise you're still a woman.)

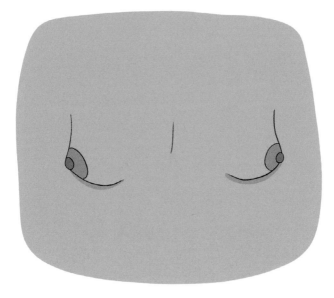

Pierced boobs

There are a whole bunch of reasons for why women want a pierced nipple, but the main ones are: they feel great (especially when touched) and they look hot. And what a whole new world of nipple jewellery they open up ... (Just make sure they are pierced by someone with the right accreditations — no one wants infected nips.)

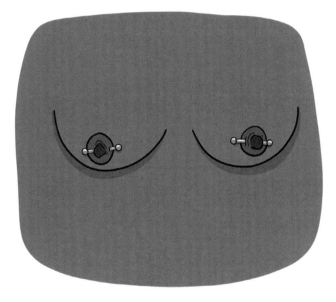

Decorated boobs

Whether you tattoo under, over, between or on your breasts, what you decide to ink can show anyone lucky enough to see your naked bosom exactly what you're all about.

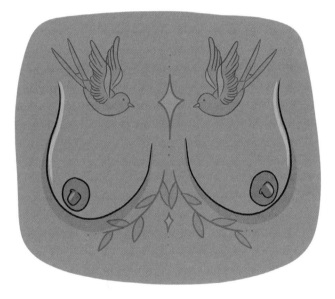

Fancy boobs

Why shouldn't the girls get their chance to dress up a little? Nipple tassels, whether for someone else or for yourself, are the ultimate fancy dress for boobs and may just awaken your inner burlesque dancer.

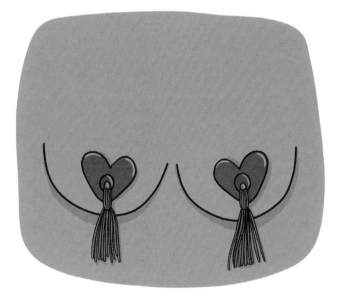

Freckly boobs

Connect the dots to find the
hidden message ... Freckles
truly are one of nature's
wonders, gifted by the sun.
Usually found on paler skin,
but can appear on any skin
tone, they are a rare and
beautiful patterning on the
skin that should be cherished.

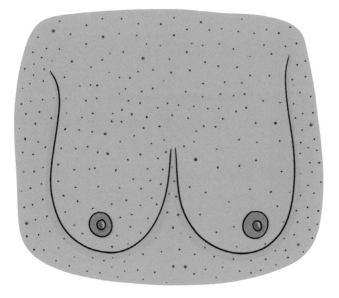

Birthmarked boobs

All breasts are exceptional and distinct, but nothing quite stamps 'unique' on a pair better than a birthmark. Whether you believe they are a kiss from the gods, a mark of destiny or simply a skin abnormality, we all agree there's something pretty special about a boob with a birthmark.

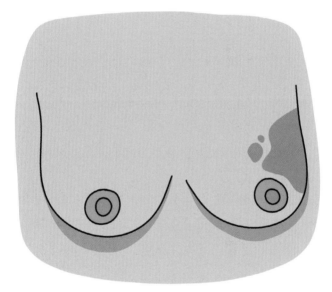

Spotty boobs

Not likely something you would choose to appear on your boobs, acne can strike anywhere and there's sometimes not a lot we can do about it. But you shouldn't let blemishes make you hide the girls away (indeed, air can help to clear the spots up!). Spots are only here on a temporary visa and your boobs are permanently wonderful.

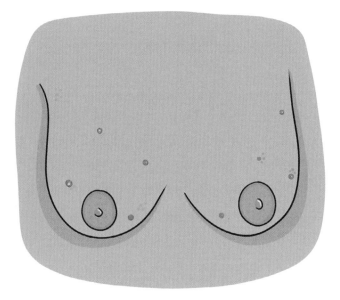

Veiny boobs

Another very natural patterning
of the breasts can be caused by
visible veins (especially common
for breastfeeding mothers).
Some women don't like theirs,
but what could be more beautiful
than a vivid blue decoration
across your bust?

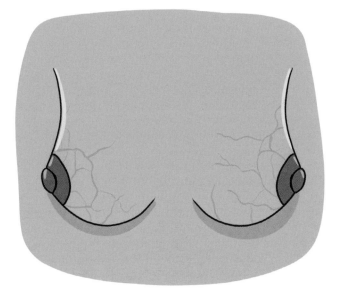

Hairy boobs

We don't all talk about it, but
pretty much all of us have hairs
around our nips — and left to
grow, they can get pretty long
too! And whether you pluck
them, snip, wax or let them
grow free is totally up to you.

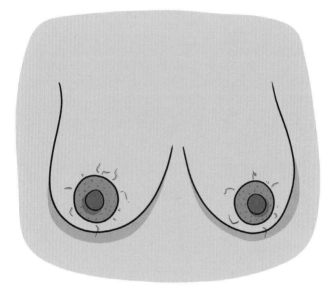

Pushed-up boobs

Whatever your breast type, sometimes it might feel nice to give the girls a little lift. Whether for a dressy night out or just to give yourself a boost on a Tuesday, there's never a bad time for a push-up bra if you're in the mood for some cleavage.

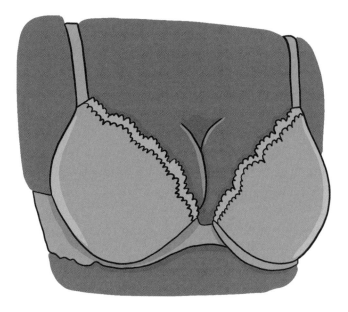

Madonnas

Unlikely to occur naturally
without some pretty specialised
surgery, this look is best
achieved with some epic bras
or fitted tops — or with the
help of Jean Paul Gaultier, if
you are Madonna. Guaranteed
to draw the eye wherever
you go, just be sure you don't
accidentally take anyone's eye
out with the pointy ends.

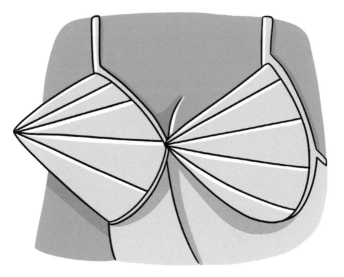

visible-nip boobs

Otherwise known as the 'smuggling peanuts' or the 'is it chilly in here or are you just happy to see me?', these may just occur when you're cold or aroused, or you might have pretty omnipresent nips. They can usually be concealed with a thicker bra or covered with silicone nap, but some people like to have theirs on display.

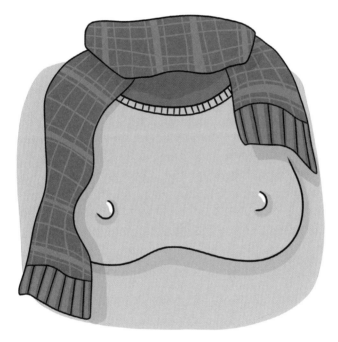

Wet boobs

It might be stating the obvious that boobs can get wet for all sorts of reasons, whether planned or unplanned, but it cannot be stressed often enough that a white top and no bra breeds the perfect condition for your entire breast to be visible. Do with that information what you will.

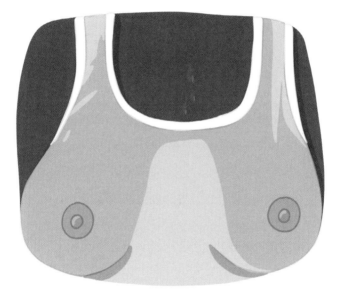

Sweaty boobs

Hopefully these only occur
for you when it's very hot,
as continually sweaty tits are
simply not comfortable (but
there are solutions if you find
yourself persistently moist).

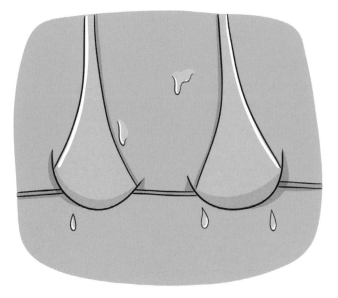

Tan-line boobs

Whether these just show up for the summer or you manage to keep up a year-long tan, usually tan lines across your boobs are seen as an undesirable outcome or celebrated as evidence of just how far your tan has come along. Of course, if you're not a fan there is an obvious way to avoid them...

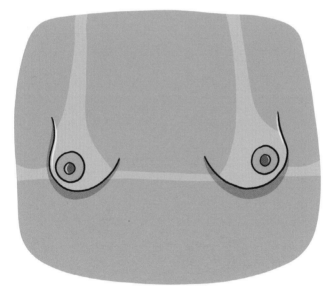

Pregnant boobs

For a lot of women, sore boobs are one of the first signs of pregnancy — often so much so that touching them is a cut-your-hand-off offence! From there they often take on a life of their own and grow to a size and shape you may not have thought they were capable of. Whether you love them or hate them, they are a sign that something pretty amazing is happening.

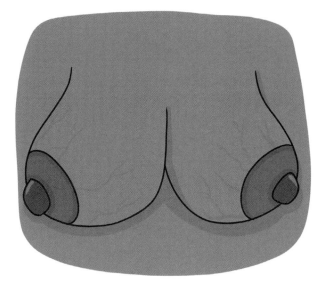

Milk-jug boobs

If your milk comes in a few days after welcoming your baby to the world, it's pretty damn uncomfortable. Bursting, straining, leaking — the early days of motherhood aren't necessarily as glowy and picture-perfect as you were expecting. But with patience, cold cabbage leaves and a stretchy nursing bra, they should calm down soon.

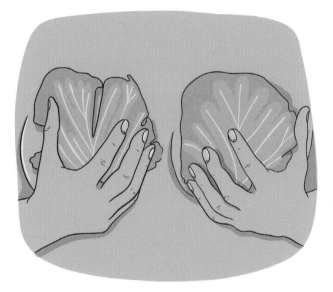

Nursing boobs

It's a pretty miraculous thing
that boobs have the potential to
sustain a life — but breastfeeding
isn't always possible. It can be
the most wonderful thing in the
world, but always remember that
FED IS BEST and bottle-feeding
is also magical.

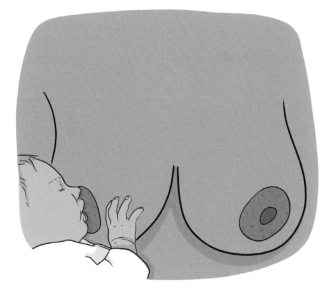

Squirty boobs

One of the not-so pleasant and sometimes very visible side effects of breastfeeding — squirty boobs. Sometimes just hearing your baby cry is enough to start a leak, but the first time they sleep for a few hours in a row — game over! You've likely leaked right out of your breast pad and are lying in sodden sheets.

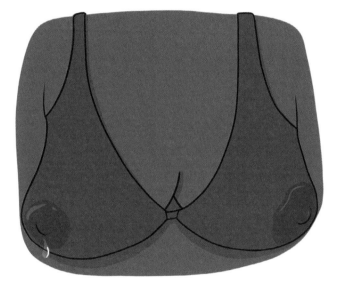

Half-fed boobs

Another breastfeeding beauty,
this breast type occurs when
your babe has fed on one side
but not deigned to have any
milk from the other. The result:
one hard, milk-filled knocker
and one soft, empty teet.

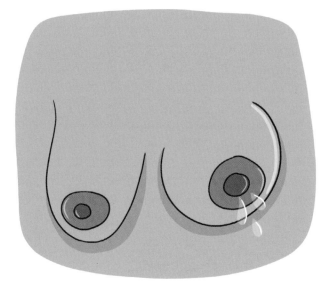

Stripey boobs

Stretch marks can occur on boobs for a number of reasons, usually after a sudden growth or reduction due to weight loss, post-pregnancy or age. They are something women might feel self-conscious about, but seen another way, these tiger stripes are a symbol of experience and the warrior woman you are.

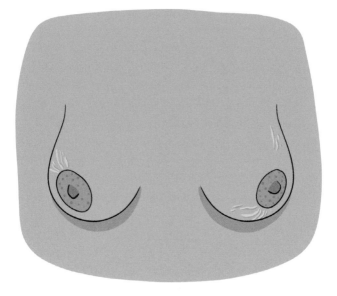

Mature boobs

Just as faces and hands age, so do our breasts go through many changes as we get older. Not only do they travel southwards and wrinkle, but they can also show age spots. While you might mourn the glory days of peachy bouncing bosoms, it can help to see your girls as symbols of a life well-lived.

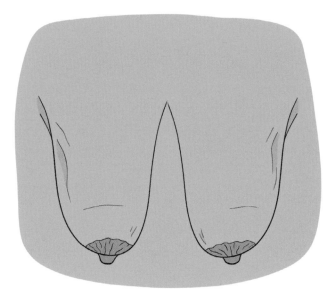

Lumpectomy boob

A cancer diagnosis can be terrifying.
From that moment on your relationship
with your breasts is likely to change,
whether you're living in the knowledge
that tumours are inside them, whether
you take meds that alter them or have
surgery to remove part or all of them.
A lumpectomy will leave a physical and
emotional scar, but that scar is also a
symbol of the price you paid to
fight cancer.

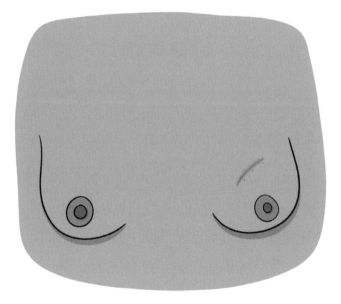

Single-mastectomy boob

A mastectomy can be life-changing and body-altering. While breasts shouldn't define us, they are a part of us, and the loss of one or both of them can be heart-breaking. No matter how much you're told that you're still beautiful (which you are), it doesn't mean you shouldn't grieve for what you've lost and how everything has changed.

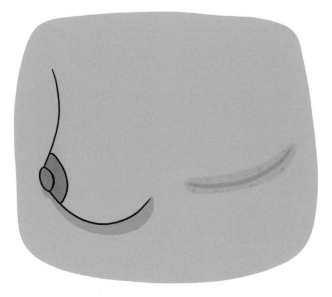

Double-mastectomy boobs

Whether preventative or curative, the decision to have surgery to remove your breasts is incredibly difficult. Only one part of your journey to fight cancer, for many women it is a painful and emotionally complicated step, but it's one that every single person who loves them will be so glad they took.

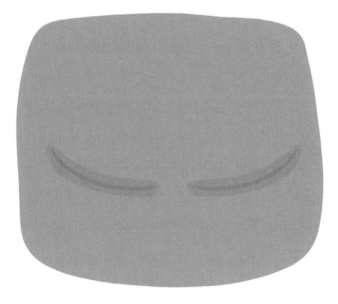

Reconstructed boobs

Every breast cancer survivor is different and will feel differently about what sits on their chest. Reconstructed breasts will never be the same as the 'real thing', so the survivor will need to develop a whole new relationship with them. But whatever they look and feel like, they are a marvel. As is the person they belong to.

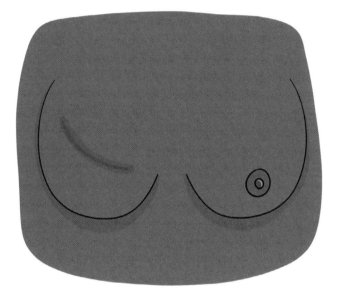

Checking your breasts

While we firmly believe every type of breast in this book is beautiful, if you notice a change in their feel or appearance (such as the emergence of veins or inverted nipples), you should get them checked out by your doctor.

Breast cancer is the most common type of cancer in the world, but there is a good chance of recovery if it is detected at any early stage. For that reason, it is vital that women check their breasts regularly, attend regular mammograms if they're eligible, and always have any changes examined by a professional.

How to check your breasts

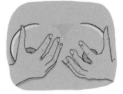

There is no wrong or right way to do this, but it's important to know how your breasts usually feel, so you can spot any changes. This may alter at different points in your menstrual cycle, but regular checking will help you to know what to expect. A good routine to follow is:

1.

Start by looking at your breasts in the mirror, both with your arms by your side and then raised. Get used to seeing the shape of your breasts and nipples, as well as what the skin typically looks like, and look out for any redness or swelling.

2.

Lying down on your back, feel your breasts, checking each with the opposite hand with firm but smooth motions. Your fingers should be kept together and your palms flat, but you will be using the pads of your fingers to feel the breast tissue. Cover the entire area, including your armpit and up to your collarbone — one of the most effective ways to check is to move your fingers up and down vertically (as if mowing a lawn). Use the same pattern every time you check them as this will ensure you're more attuned to changes.

3.

Repeat this standing up — it's usually easiest in the shower with soap to keep the movement smooth.

HarperCollins*Publishers*
1 London Bridge Street
London SE1 9GF

www.harpercollins.co.uk

HarperCollins*Publishers*
1st Floor, Watermarque Building, Ringsend Road
Dublin 4, Ireland

First published by HarperCollins*Publishers* 2022

10 9 8 7 6 5 4 3 2 1

Text by Anna Mrowiec © HarperCollins*Publishers* 2022

Illustrations by Louisa Foley © HarperCollins*Publishers* 2022

HarperCollins*Publishers* asserts the moral right to be identified as the author
of this work

A catalogue record of this book is available from the British Library

ISBN 978-0-00-854666-3

Printed and bound in Latvia by PNB

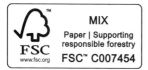

This book is produced from independently certified FSC™ paper
to ensure responsible forest management.

For more information visit: www.harpercollins.co.uk/green

Changes to look out for

You should consult with your doctor if you notice any of the following changes:

- A difference in the shape, size or outline of your breast
- A new swelling or lump(s) in the breast or armpit
- Any change in the position or appearance of your nipple
- A change in the feel or look of your breast, such as redness, a rash, dimpling or puckering
- Discharge from either of your nipples
- Pain or discomfort in one breast

While these changes could occur for many reasons, most of which are not serious, it is always best to see a doctor to be safe.